DK Natural Care Library

VITAMINS

BALANCING BODY & MIND

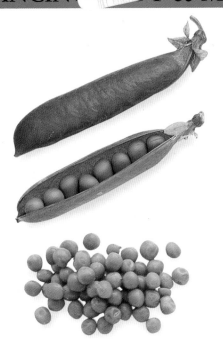

By STEPHANIE PEDERSEN

DORLING KINDERSLEY PUBLISHING, INC.

www.dk.com

CONTENTS

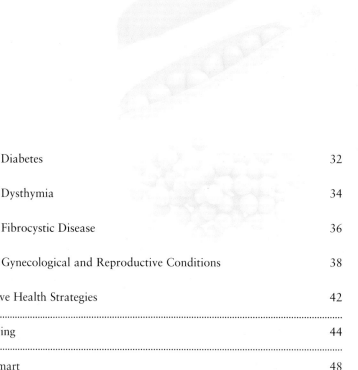

WHAT IS VITAMIN B?

The term "vitamin B" actually refers to "vitamin B-complex," a group of eight closely related but chemically distinct vitamins that frequently work together to maintain health. Some B vitamins are referred to by their "B name," while others are better known by their chemical name. The B-complex vitamins are vitamin B_1 (thiamin), vitamin B_2 (riboflavin), vitamin B_3 (niacin), vitamin B_5 (pantothenic acid), vitamin B_6 (pyridoxine), vitamin B_7 (biotin), vitamin B_9 (folic acid or folate), and vitamin B_{12} (cobalamin). Their combined functions include maintaining skin and muscle tone, enhancing immune and nervous system functions, promoting cell growth and division, encouraging proper brain function, and sustaining the health of eyes, hair, liver, and mouth.

The B-complex vitamins share other characteristics. All are water-soluble, meaning that instead of storing unused amounts of these vitamins, the body excretes whatever it doesn't use. All are poorly absorbed by the elderly, making adequate intake of B-complex vitamins important as humans age. All B vitamins should be taken together, although taking two or three times more of one or several of the individual B vitamins is common for particular disorders. All B-complex vitamins are found to a certain extent in brewer's yeast, brown rice, green leafy vegetables, eggs, fish, legumes, nuts, organ meats, soy products, and whole grains. Because they are frequently found together in foods, a deficiency of one B vitamin often means a deficiency of several or all of the B vitamins.

As similar as the B-complex vitamins are, however, they are not identical. Continue reading to learn more about each individual vitamin.

ALL TOGETHER NOW
For individuals who need help in getting enough vitamin B-complex, supplements are important. But to take eight pills at one time can be daunting. A better option is a vitamin B-complex supplement containing all eight vitamins. Look for a product that contains at least the minimum RDA (recommended daily allowances) for each separate nutrient.

HOW MUCH DO I TAKE?

How many times have you stood in front of the vitamin shelves in your local health food store or pharmacy and compared labels? And how many times have you wondered why one brand offers 60 mg of vitamin C when another boasts 750 mg of vitamin C? Or why another product has 180 mcg of folate when a competing brand features 400 mcg of the same nutrient? And perhaps more importantly, which one is better? When it comes to dosages, there is no magic number. Minimum requirements for nutrients are set by a government board called The Food and Nutrition Board of the National Research Council. These numbers are the recommended daily allowances (RDA) needed to avoid nutritional deficiency diseases such as beriberi, rickets, or scurvy. However, many researchers, medical experts, and health authorities believe that the body needs much higher levels of vitamins for optimum health. And in the presence of illness, pollution, prescription medication, or stress, the body may need still higher levels. For this reason, throughout this book, we suggest a range of vitamin dosages. To determine the best level for you, consult your physician.

VITAMIN B₁ (THIAMIN)

Up until 1930, thousands of people each year died of a central nervous system disease called beriberi. The disease damaged nerves, leaving victims mentally impaired, crippled, paralyzed, or dead. In 1930, scientists discovered a substance in food that prevented the disease. The substance was named thiamin, also known as vitamin B_1, and soon commercially milled flours were enriched with the vitamin.

Vitamin B_1 enhances circulation, assists in blood formation, aids in carbohydrate metabolism, and is needed to produce hydrochloric acid, which helps digest food. The vitamin also helps convert excess blood glucose into stored fat. It maintains proper nerve-impulse transmission, optimizes cognitive activity, and maintains brain function. The vitamin also maintains the muscles of the intestines, stomach, and heart. Thiamin additionally has an antioxidant effect, protecting the body from the harmful effects of alcohol, pollutants, and smoking.

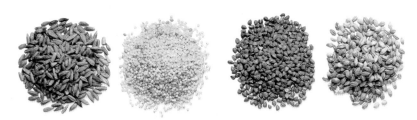

• **Minimum Recommended Dosage:** Men, 1.5 mg; women, 1.1 mg; pregnant women, 1.5 mg. Thiamin is considered nontoxic even in high doses.

• **Deficiency Symptoms:** Appetite loss, constipation, fatigue, forgetfulness, gastrointestinal disturbances, irregular heartbeat, irritability, labored breathing, muscle atrophy, nervousness, numbness in hands and feet, poor coordination, weakness, and weight loss. Severe vitamin B_1 deficiency can cause beriberi.

• **Food Sources:** Brewer's yeast, brown rice, egg yolks, fish, legumes, peanuts, peas, pork, wheat germ, and whole grains.

• **Special Needs:** Individuals who take antibiotics or sulfa drugs, are on oral contraceptives, drink alcohol daily, eat a diet high in simple carbohydrates, or exercise heavily each day have increased needs for vitamin B_1.

• **Cautions:** Vitamin B_1 is best absorbed when ingested with other B vitamins.

VITAMIN B$_2$ (RIBOFLAVIN)

Although it is rare today, at one time ariboflavinosis was often seen among individuals with limited diets. Characterized by eye disorders, impaired mental functioning, inflammation of the mouth and tongue, mouth sores, skin lesions, sore throat, and weakness, the disease was discovered to be caused by a deficiency of riboflavin, hence the disease's name.

Like other members of the B-vitamin family, riboflavin helps the body metabolize carbohydrates, fats, and proteins. Also known as vitamin B$_2$, the nutrient is fundamental in red blood cell formation, antibody production, and cell respiration. It facilitates the utilization of oxygen by the tissues of the skin, mucous membranes (including the mucous membranes of the digestive tract), nails, and hair. The vitamin is needed for the body to metabolize niacin, another B vitamin. It is also necessary for healthy eye tissue and alleviates eye fatigue, and it is important in the prevention and treatment of cataracts. Vitamin B$_2$ is especially critical during pregnancy to help promote normal fetal growth.

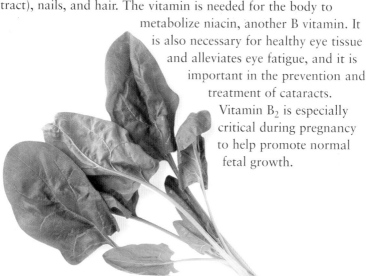

• **Minimum Recommended Dosage:** Men, 1.7 mg; women, 1.3 mg; pregnant women, 1.6 mg; lactating women, 1.8 mg. Because the body cannot absorb large amounts of vitamin B_2 at one time, there is no known toxicity level for this vitamin.

• **Deficiency Symptoms:** Cracks at the corners of the mouth, dermatitis, dizziness, hair loss, insomnia, itchy or burning eyes, light sensitivity, mouth sores, impaired thinking, inflammation of the tongue, and rashes.

• **Food Sources:** Most plant and animal foods contain some vitamin B_2. The best sources are almonds, broccoli, cheese, green leafy vegetables, egg yolks, fish, legumes, milk, organ meats, poultry, soy products, spinach, whole grains, and yogurt. Interestingly, it has been estimated that up to one-third of North American vitamin B_2 intake is from dairy products.

• **Special Needs:** Individuals who take antibiotics or oral contraceptives, drink alcohol daily, or exercise heavily each day have increased needs for vitamin B_2. Because they do not metabolize the vitamin efficiently, elderly people also need higher levels of vitamin B_2.

• **Cautions:** Nervousness and rapid heartbeat have been reported with daily dosages of 10 mg. When taken in doses above 100 mg, vitamin B_2 can cause photosensitivity.

VITAMIN B₃ (NIACIN)

Pellagra was once a relatively common disease in the United States. Characterized by anxiety, chronic diarrhea, dermatitis, dizziness, headaches, progressive dementia, weakness, and weight loss, pellagra was most often observed among poor individuals, especially those who existed on a corn-based diet. Not until 1942, however, was the nutrient responsible for preventing pellagra discovered. Named niacin, or vitamin B₃, the vitamin—which is not found in corn—was added to enriched flour and other commercially made products, making the disease virtually nonexistent today.

Niacin contributes to more than 50 vital bodily processes. Like other B vitamins, it helps the body metabolize carbohydrates, fats, and proteins and is necessary for the production of hydrochloric acid, which is used in food digestion. The vitamin is involved in the normal secretion of bile and stomach fluids. It is necessary for red blood cell formation and blood circulation, lowers cholesterol and is a vasodilator. It assists in the maintenance of skin, nerves, and blood vessels. Vitamin B₃ regulates blood sugar levels, is needed in the synthesis of sex hormones, and detoxifies the body of certain drugs and chemicals. It is necessary for normal mental functioning.

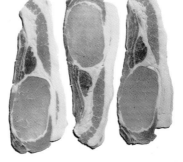

• **Minimum Recommended Dosage:** Men, 19 mg; women, 15 mg; pregnant women, 17 mg; lactating women, 20 mg. Vitamin B_3 is toxic in large amounts. However, because of the extreme nausea that accompanies large doses of niacin, there are few reported cases of individuals taking enough niacin to overdose.

• **Deficiency Symptoms:** Depression, dizziness, fatigue, halitosis, headaches, indigestion, insomnia, limb pains, loss of appetite, low blood sugar, mouth sores, muscular weakness, and skin eruptions.

• **Food Sources:** Brewer's yeast, broccoli, carrots, cheese, corn flour, dandelion greens, dates, eggs, fish, milk, peanuts, pork, potatoes, tomatoes, and wheat germ.

• **Special Needs:** Individuals who drink alcohol daily have increased needs for vitamin B_3. Because they do not metabolize the vitamin efficiently, elderly people and individuals with hyperthyroidism also need higher levels of vitamin B_3.

• **Cautions:** Dosages of niacin over 50 to 100 mg can cause temporary flushing in some individuals. Taking more than 500 mg daily for several months at a time may cause liver damage. For that reason, people with hepatitis or other liver disease should consult a doctor before taking large amounts of niacin.

VITAMIN B$_5$ (PANTOTHENIC ACID)

Vitamin B$_5$, also known as pantothenic acid, is essential for growth, reproduction, and normal physiological functions. It is required by all cells in the body and is involved in more than 100 different metabolic functions, including energy metabolism of carbohydrates, proteins, and lipids, the synthesis of lipids, neuro-transmitters, steroid hormones, porphyrins, and hemoglobin. The vitamin helps build red blood cells, assists in making bile, and is necessary for the normal functioning of the gastrointestinal tract. It is also a stamina enhancer and has been found to be helpful in treating depression.

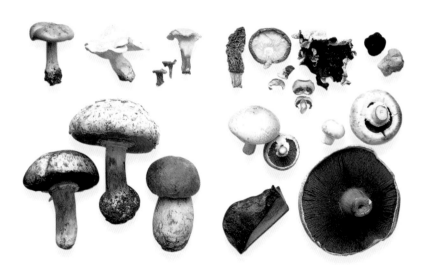

• **Minimum Recommended Dosage:** 4 to 7 mg. The average American diet provides between 3 and 6 mg of vitamin B_5.

• **Deficiency Symptoms:** Vitamin B_5 deficiency is extremely rare and is likely only to occur with starvation. Deficiency symptoms include fatigue, headache, and nausea.

• **Food Sources:** Most plant and animal foods contain some vitamin B_5. In fact, the root *pan*, in pantothenic acid, is the Greek term for "everywhere," indicating this vitamin's abundance. Natural sources include avocado, brewer's yeast, eggs, beans, brown rice, corn, lentils, mushrooms, nuts, organ meats, peas, pork, saltwater fish, soybeans, sweet potatoes, and wheat germ.

• **Special Needs:** None.

• **Cautions:** There is no known toxicity level for this vitamin. However, doses above 10 mg can cause diarrhea in some individuals.

VITAMIN B$_6$ (PYRIDOXINE)

Although vitamin B$_6$ isn't as talked about as some of its B-vitamin cousins, it's among the busiest nutrient within the B-complex. It is involved in more bodily functions than almost any other single nutrient. Like other B vitamins, vitamin B$_6$ helps metabolize carbohydrates, fats, and proteins. Also called pyridoxine, the nutrient supports normal immune-system, nervous-system, and mental functions. The vitamin is essential for nerve impulse transmission within the brain and is necessary for antibody production. It maintains the body's sodium-potassium balance, aids in the formation of red blood cells, and helps synthesize RNA and DNA. It protects the heart by inhibiting the formation of homocysteine, a toxic chemical that attacks the heart muscle and contributes to cholesterol deposits around the heart. The vitamin also assists the body in absorbing and metabolizing other B vitamins.

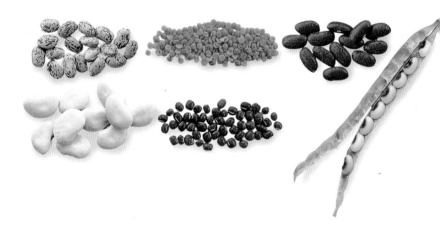

• **Minimum Recommended Dosage:** Men, 2 mg; women, 1.6 mg; pregnant women, 2.2 mg.

• **Deficiency Symptoms:** Vitamin B_6 deficiency is rare. Symptoms include depression, fatigue, flaky skin, headache, insomnia, irritability, mouth sores, muscle weakness, and nausea.

• **Food Sources:** Avocados, bananas, beans, blackstrap molasses, brown rice, carrots, corn, fish, legumes, nuts, poultry, soybeans, sunflower seeds, tempeh, walnuts, and wheat germ.

• **Special Needs:** Individuals taking antidepressants, cortisone drugs, diuretics, hormone replacement therapy, or oral contraceptives have increased needs for vitamin B_6. Because they do not metabolize the vitamin efficiently, elderly people and individuals with celiac disease and diabetes also need higher levels of vitamin B_6.

• **Cautions:** When taken for three months or more, levels of 2,000 to 5,000 mg can cause diarrhea, insomnia, and/or numbness in the hands and feet.

VITAMIN B₇ (BIOTIN)

Biotin, or vitamin B_7, is another B vitamin with varied duties. Best known by many people as a moisturizing agent in shampoos, conditioners, and skin creams, biotin is essential to numerous body processes. As with other B vitamins, biotin allows the body to metabolize carbohydrates, fats, and proteins. It aids in cell growth, is necessary for fatty acid production, and must be present for the body to metabolize other B vitamins. Biotin also promotes normal function of the sweat glands, nerve tissue, and bone marrow, and helps relieve muscle pain.

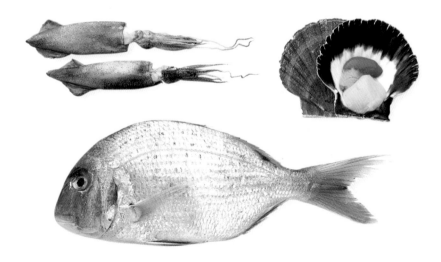

- **Minimum Recommended Dosage:** 30 to 100 mcg.

- **Deficiency Symptoms:** Though biotin deficiency is rare, it can lead to fatigue, loss of appetite, depression, hair loss, lethargy, muscle pain, nausea, and skin rashes.

- **Food Sources:** Most foods contain some amount of biotin. It is found in highest concentrations, however, in beef, brewer's yeast, broccoli, egg yolks, kidneys, milk, nuts, poultry, saltwater fish, soybeans, sunflower seeds, sweet potatoes, and whole grains.

- **Special Needs:** Individuals taking antibiotics, anticonvulsants, or sulfa drugs have increased needs for vitamin B_7. Individuals who consume saccharin or raw egg whites regularly—each of which contains a protein called avidin, which blocks the body's absorption of biotin—need extra vitamin B_7.

- **Cautions:** Current research has not revealed a toxic dosage for biotin. In tests, oral and intravenous doses of up to 20 mg of biotin have not produced toxicity in humans.

VITAMIN B₉(FOLIC ACID)

Folic acid has received much attention lately for its role in preventing low birth weightin infants and premature birth, as well as neural tube defects, such as spina bifida and anencephaly, in developing fetuses. Known also as folate or vitamin B_9, the vitamin is necessary for healthy nervous system functioning. Like other B vitamins, folic acid aids in the formation of red blood cells, the metabolism of protein, and the synthesis of DNA and RNA. It is also important for cell division and replication. The vitamin helps manufacture white blood cells and is necessary for immune-system functioning.

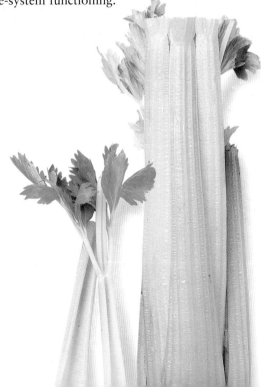

• **Minimum Recommended Dosage:** Men, 200 mcg; women, 180 mcg; women of childbearing age, 400 mcg.

• **Deficiency Symptoms:** Appetite loss, diarrhea, fatigue, insomnia, pallor, and a red, inflamed tongue. Extreme folic acid deficiency—often seen in alcoholics—can cause folic acid anemia, characterized by malformation and reduction of red blood cells.

• **Food Sources:** Apricots, asparagus, avocados, barley, Brussels sprouts, dried beans, brewer's yeast, brown rice, cantaloupe, celery, eggs, fish, green leafy vegetables, lentils, mushrooms, nuts, oranges, organ meats, peas, root vegetables, seeds, some fortified breakfast cereals, tempeh, wheat bran, and wheat germ.

• **Special Needs:** Individuals who drink alcohol daily or who take oral contraceptives have increased needs for vitamin B_9. Due to the risk of infant birth defects associated with low levels of folic acid, it is recommended that all women of childbearing age get 400 mcg of folic acid daily to ensure that any unplanned pregnancy produces a healthy infant.

• **Cautions:** A toxic level of folic acid has not been established, but daily doses above 400 mcg can mask symptoms of pernicious anemia and counteract anti epileptic drugs.

VITAMIN B₁₂ (COBALAMIN)

Vitamin B_{12}, also known as cobalamin, is best known for its role in preventing anemia. The vitamin works with folic acid to help form and regulate red blood cells. It also helps the body absorb and utilize iron. It aids in cell formation and cellular longevity and is critical in producing RNA and DNA and maintaining fertility. Just like other B vitamins, cobalamin helps metabolize carbohydrates, fats, and proteins. It is essential in producing myelin, a fatty substance that forms a protective sheath around nerves. Vitamin B_{12} is also linked to the production of acetylcholine, a neurotransmitter that assists memory and learning.

Unlike other B vitamins, vitamin B_{12} takes several hours to be absorbed by the digestive tract. While excess vitamin B_{12} is excreted in the urine, a small "backup" supply is stored for three to five years in the liver.

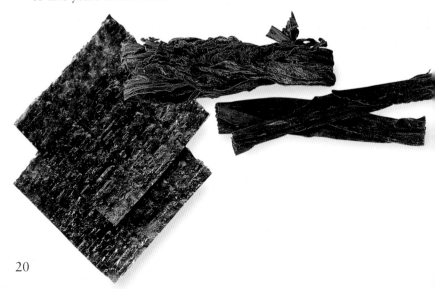

- **Minimum Recommended Dosage:** Adults, 2 mcg; pregnant women, 2.2 mcg.

- **Deficiency Symptoms:** While deficiency is rare, individuals who do not eat animal products are at risk unless they fortify their diets with plant sources of B_{12}, such as brewer's yeast, sea vegetables, and tempeh. Symptoms include back pain, body odor, constipation, dizziness, fatigue, moodiness, numbness and tingling in the arms and legs, ringing in the ears, muscle weakness, tongue inflammation, and weight loss.

- **Food Sources:** Brewer's yeast, dairy products, eggs, organ meats, seafood, sea vegetables, and tempeh.

- **Special Needs:** Individuals taking anticoagulant drugs, anti gout medication, or potassium supplements have increased needs for vitamin B_{12}. Individuals, including vegetarians, who do not eat foods that contain vitamin B_{12}, need vitamin B_{12} supplements. Because they have difficulty absorbing the vitamin, the elderly and people with AIDS also have increased needs for vitamin B_{12}.

- **Cautions:** No toxic effects have been reported when up to 100 mg a day are consumed.

CONDITIONS AND DOSES

ACNE

❒ **Symptoms:** Acne is an inflammatory skin disorder. It occurs when hormones stimulate the overproduction of keratin and sebum, which in turn get caught in the skin's pores, causing blackheads. Often bacteria mixes with the excess keratin and sebum, resulting in infected whiteheads and cystlike pustules. While acne generally affects the face, it also occurs on the neck, chest, and back, and can be mild to severe.

❒ **How Vitamin B_5 and Vitamin B_6 Can Help:** American research has found that B-complex vitamins B_5 and B_6 help heal acne. Both vitamin B_5 and vitamin B_6 are necessary for healthy skin cells. Both help reduce inflammation in individual pustules, regenerate healthy epidermal tissue, and produce infection-fighting white blood cells—which in turn consume invading bacteria. Furthermore, blood tests have found that many people with acne are deficient in Vitamin B_6, a vitamin that has proved to be especially effective in diminishing premenstrual acne flare-ups in women. While it is not known exactly how the vitamin does this, it is believed to help the body balance hormone levels.

❒ **Dosages:** Take 25 to 50 mg of vitamin B-complex once or twice a day; plus an additional 5 to 10 mg of vitamin B_5 three times a day; and an additional 10 to 20 mg of vitamin B_6 three times a day.

TOPICALLY SPEAKING

Topical creams are a popular treatment for acne. These products usually contain ingredients such as glycolic acid, salicylic acid, sulfur, or benzoyl peroxide. Recent studies, however, have found certain B vitamins are also effective when used topically to fight pimples. In one trial, acne patients used a cream containing 20 percent vitamin B_5, applying it from four to six times a day. Test subjects with moderate acne saw near-complete relief within two months; individuals with severe acne saw improvement after six months. Niacin, also known as vitamin B_3, is another B-complex vitamin found to substantially help people with acne. In a double-blind trial lasting two months, test subjects applied a topical gel containing four percent niacin twice a day. After two months, all had seen improvement.

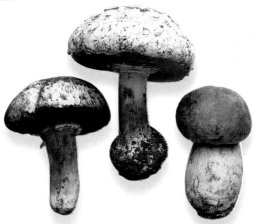

CONDITIONS AND DOSES

ASTHMA

❏ **Symptoms:** Asthma is an inflammation of the airways. It is caused by an allergic reaction and is estimated to affect between 10 million and 14 million Americans. Although not all sufferers are allergic to the same substances, some common triggers are animal dander, dust mites, mold spores, and pollen. When a trigger is inhaled, the body's antibodies react with the allergen, producing allergen-suppressing histamine and other chemicals. Also, chest muscles constrict, the bronchial lining swells, and the body creates more mucus, thus causing difficulty breathing, coughing (sometimes accompanied by mucus), painless tightness in the chest, and wheezing.

❏ **How Vitamin B_6 Can Help:** Several studies have found that individuals with asthma are commonly lacking vitamin B_6. While the vitamin cannot cure asthma, it does help the body produce antibodies, which in turn help inhibit allergens. Vitamin B_6 also strengthens the immune system, making it more efficient at fending off allergen attacks.

❏ **Dosages:** As a preventative, take 25 to 50 mg of vitamin B-complex once or twice a day, plus an additional 10 to 20 mg of vitamin B_6 three times a day.

MISERY LOVES COMPANY

If you suffer from asthma, you're not alone. According to the American Lung Association, since 1982, the prevalence of asthma in the United States increased by 49 percent; among children under age 18, the rate rose 78.6 percent. More breath taking statistics: More than 4,000 people die each year from serious asthma attacks.

THE HYDROCHLORIC ACID CONNECTION

While studies have recently confirmed the link between low vitamin B_6 levels and asthma symptoms, science has long known that one of the vitamin's duties is to help create hydrochloric acid, a stomach acid necessary for digestion. What do these seemingly unrelated things have in common? Research has found that asthmatic children regularly test positive for low levels of hydrochloric acid in thje stomach, thus strengthening the connection between vitamin B_6 deficiency and asthma.

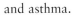

CONDITIONS AND DOSES

CANKER SORES

❐ **Symptoms:** It's not known exactly what causes canker sores, or aphthous ulcers, as they're also known—though irritation from dental work, nutritional deficiencies, a poorly functioning immune system, and stress have all been implicated. These small, painful ulcers can appear singly or in clusters on the gums, insides of the cheeks, insides of the lips, or on the tongue. Each ulcer contains a coagulated mixture of fluid, bacteria, and white blood cells.

❐ **How Vitamin B_1, Vitamin B_2, and Vitamin B_6 Can Help:** Several reports have found a surprisingly high incidence of vitamin B_1, B_2, and B_6 deficiency among people with recurrent canker sores. These vitamins are responsible for maintaining healthy tissue and protecting mucous membranes.

❐ **Dosages:** As a preventative or a treatment, take 25 to 50 mg of vitamin B-complex once or twice a day, plus an additional daily dose of 300 mg of vitamin B_1, 20 mg of vitamin B_2, and 150 mg of vitamin B_6. **Note:** Vitamin B_6 has been shown to be safe in amounts of 200 to 500 mg per day. However, if you experience numbness in the hands or feet, stop taking the individual vitamin B_6 supplement. Lactating women should not take more than 100 mg of vitamin B_6 a day.

GINGIVITIS

❒ **Symptoms:** Caused by deposits of plaque along the gum line, gingivitis is a painless condition characterized by swollen, soft, red gums that bleed easily during brushing and flossing. Certain drugs, such as phenytoin—a drug used for seizure disorders and neuralgia—can increase the production of plaque, thus increasing one's odds of developing gingivitis. If left untreated, gingivitis can worsen into periodontitis and tooth loss.

❒ **How Vitamin B_9 Can Help:** Vitamin B_9 cannot cure gingivitis—only a professional dental cleaning and regular brushing and flossing can do that. But when used as a companion strategy to professional and home dental care, the vitamin has been shown to reduce inflammation and help regenerate healthy gum tissue.

❒ **Dosages:** Take 25 to 50 mg of vitamin B-complex once or twice a day, plus an additional 100 mcg of vitamin B_9 three times per day. In severe cases, ask your dentist about folic acid mouth rinses. Rinse with a 0.1 percent dental solution of folic acid twice a day.

CONDITIONS AND DOSES

CARPAL TUNNEL SYNDROME

❏ **Symptoms:** The carpal tunnel is a passageway through the wrist that protects those nerves and tendons that link the arm and hand. When the tissue that constitutes the tunnel becomes inflamed through repetitive motion, carpal tunnel syndrome occurs. The result is numbness or tingling in the hand and fingers and pain in the wrist that may shoot up into the forearm or down into the fingers.

❏ **How Vitamin B_6 Can Help:** Vitamin B_6 is one of the most frequently used nutritional treatments for carpal tunnel syndrome. And with good reason: The vitamin has been shown both to protect carpal tunnel tissue and reduce inflammation in the carpal tunnel, thus preventing the syndrome and relieving symptoms in established cases. Furthermore, research has found that many people with carpal tunnel syndrome have vitamin B_6 deficiencies.

❏ **Dosages:** Take 25 to 50 mg of vitamin B-complex once or twice a day, plus an additional 50 to 100 mg of vitamin B_6 three times per day. Mild results will be seen within a month, with more dramatic results occurring within two to three months. **Note:** Vitamin B_6 has been shown to be safe in amounts of 200 to 500 mg per day. However, if you experience numbness in the hands or feet, stop taking the individual vitamin B_6 supplement. Lactating women should not take more than 100 mg of vitamin B_6 a day.

A SHOT IN THE ARM

A bursa is a saclike membrane that acts as a cushion between the bone and fibrous tissues of the muscles and tendons. Its job is to facilitate movement by limiting friction. When a bursa becomes inflamed through repeated physical activity, the result is bursitis. Symptoms include pain and swelling in a joint, usually the elbow, hip, knee, shoulder, or big toe.

Conventional treatment for this painful condition is cortisone injected directly into the affected area. Yet cortisone, a steroid that reduces inflammation, has numerous long-term side effects, including bone loss and kidney damage. Fortunately for bursitis sufferers, research has discovered a more risk-free option: injections of high doses of vitamin B_{12} or a combination of B_{12} and B_3. Studies show that both options not only relieve symptoms and reduce inflammation, they also decrease the calcification deposits that sometimes occur in chronically inflamed bursa. While it isn't understood exactly how vitamin B_{12} and vitamin B_3 relieve bursitis symptoms, studies have found that taking large doses of the two vitamins orally does not have the same beneficial effect as the injections, which allow the affected area to utilize the entire dose of the vitamin. In contrast, oral intake dispenses the vitamin throughout the body for the whole body's use.

CONDITIONS AND DOSES

OSTEOARTHRITIS

❒ **Symptoms:** Osteoarthritis, also known simply as arthritis, is one of the most common disorders known to humans, affecting up to 80 percent of all individuals over the age of 60. Caused by simple wear and tear on a joint, arthritis is considered a degenerative disease. Symptoms include mild to moderately severe pain in a joint during or after use, discomfort in a joint during a weather change, swelling in an affected joint, and loss of flexibility in an affected joint.

❒ **How Vitamin B$_3$ Can Help:** American and Canadian research has found that high doses of vitamin B$_3$, or niacin, as it's also called, can help lessen osteoarthritis symptoms by increasing joint mobility and improving muscle strength. It is believed that the vitamin works by increasing blood circulation to affected joints and helping to regenerate healthy new tissue.

❒ **Dosages:** Take 25 to 50 mg of vitamin B-complex once or twice a day, day, plus an additional 200 to 250 mg of vitamin B$_3$ three times a day. Mild results will be seen within a month, with more dramatic results occurring within three or four months. **Note:** Dosages of niacin over 50 to 100 mg can cause temporary flushing in some individuals. Taking more than 500 mg daily for several months at a time may cause liver damage. For that reason, people with hepatitis or other liver disease should consult a doctor before taking large amounts of niacin.

THE FOLIC ACID FOLLIES

Pregnancy is not the time to begin experimenting with large doses of different vitamins. It is imperative, however, that you get enough nutrients during this time to support a quickly-developing fetus. One of the most talked-about vitamins for fetal development is folic acid, also called vitamin B_9 and folate, which is famous for its role in the development of genetic material such as RNA and DNA. Because a large number of pregnancies in the United States are unplanned, it is important for women to get enough folic acid throughout their childbearing years—thus ensuring that any unintentional pregnancy will be a healthy one. The recommended daily dose of folic acid during childbearing years and pregnancy is 400 to 800 mcg per day. Here's how the vitamin can help:

• Deficiencies of folic acid have been linked in studies to low birth weight in infants. In one study, folic acid supplements in pregnant women improved birth weight and decreased the incidence of fetal growth retardation and maternal infections.

• Research has linked low folic acid intake to neural tube defects, such as spina bifida. Women have been reported to lower their risk of having a child with spina bifida by 72 percent if they take folic acid supplements prior to and during pregnancy.

• Taking one of folic acid's B-complex cousins, niacin, in the first trimester has been positively correlated with higher birth-weight, longer length, and larger head circumference, all signs of healthier infants. Pregnant women should take a daily dose of at least 17 mcg of niacin—or vitamin B_3, as it's also called.

CONDITIONS AND DOSES

DIABETES

❐ **Symptoms:** To understand diabetes, it helps to know something about the pancreas. The organ—long, thin, and situated behind the stomach—is responsible for regulating the body's use of glucose. To do so, the pancreas creates a number of chemicals, including insulin. When blood glucose levels begin to rise, it is insulin's job to prod muscle and fat cells to absorb whatever glucose they need for future activities; the liver stores any surplus. Some individuals, however, either do not produce enough insulin or their body resists whatever insulin is produced, thus necessitating an outside source is required. Either way, the result is the same: diabetes—specifically, diabetes type 1 and diabetes type 2.

Type 1, or juvenile-onset diabetes, typically affects children and young adults and is genetically linked. Type 2, or adult-onset diabetes, occurs in adults and is linked to obesity. Symptoms of both types include blurred vision, fatigue, frequent bladder infections, increased appetite, increased thirst, increased urination, nausea, skin infections, vaginitis, and vomiting. If not treated, diabetes type 1 and type 2 can cause blood vessel damage, gangrene, heart attack, kidney damage, nerve damage, stroke, and vision problems.

❐ **How Vitamin B_7 and Vitamin B_{12} Can Help:** Vitamin B_7, also known as biotin, helps the body metabolize glucose, making it a popularly prescribed vitamin for diabetics. Vitamin B_{12} has been shown to prevent or decrease nerve damage in diabetics.

❑ **Dosages:** Take 25 to 50 mg of vitamin B-complex once or twice a day; plus an additional 30 to 50 mcg of vitamin B_7 three times a day; and an additional 2 mcg of vitamin B_{12} three times a day.

EAT YOUR WAY TO HEALTH

When you're diabetic, what you do and don't eat immediately becomes important. One wrong bite can send glucose levels soaring—or plummeting. Underscoring the importance of diet is a recent study of 21 diabetics with diabetic nerve damage. The results of the study, reported in several medical journals—including the *American Journal of Clinical Nutrition,* the *American Journal of Public Health,* and the *Journal of Nutritional Medicine*—indicate that when fed a vegan diet (no meat, dairy, or eggs), all test subjects experienced some pain reduction, while 17 experienced a complete disappearance of pain. Vegans eat less fat and less protein than meat eaters, who often get much more protein than needed to maintain health. Reducing fat and protein intake has been found to reduce the kidney damage caused by diabetes and to improve glucose tolerance.

CONDITIONS AND DOSES

DYSTHYMIA

❑ **Symptoms:** Translated from the Greek, dysthymia means "bad mood." In medical-speak, however, the term refers to mild to moderate depression. The condition often begins with no apparent trigger, though it can also develop from adjustment disorder. Symptoms can include change in appetite, decreased self-esteem, grief, helplessness, impaired daily functioning, irritability, loss of interest in once enjoyable activities, inappropriate guilt, lethargy, neglect of physical appearance, malaise, self-reproach, sense of doom, sleep disturbances, slowed physical and mental responses, social withdrawal, and thoughts of suicide.

❑ **How Vitamin B_6 and Vitamin B_9 Can Help:** Research has shown that many depressed people are low in vitamin B_6, a vitamin needed for transmission of nerve impulses in the brain. In one trial, 20 mg of vitamin B_6, given twice a day, was shown to alleviate symptoms of depression. Another B vitamin that has been shown to help treat depression is folic acid. Also called vitamin B_9, the nutrient is necessary for healthy brain and nerve functioning and has been shown in tests to be low in a large percentage of depressed people.

❑ **Dosages:** Take 25 to 50 mg of vitamin B-complex once or twice a day; plus an additional 10 to 20 mg of vitamin B_6 three times a day; and an additional 100 to 200 mcg of folic acid three times a day. You should begin seeing mild changes in mood after a week and more dramatic improvement after four weeks.

MIGRAINE MEDICINE

Also called a vascular headache, a migraine is an extremely painful headaches that occur when cerebral blood vessels constrict, allowing less blood to reach the brain. The one constant symptom is severe head pain—often so extreme that individuals become nauseated and vomit. The pain typically begins on one side of the head and may gradually spread and throb.

Migraines are usually preceded by several warning signs. Two to eight hours before the migraine occurs, there may be cravings for sweets, elation, drowsiness, intense thirst, and irritability. About 15 to 30 minutes before the migraine occurs there is the classic aura, a group of signs that can include blank spots within the field of vision, dizziness, sparkling flashes of light, temporary numbness or paralysis of one side of the body, and zigzag lines that cross the field of vision. It is not known why some people get migraines, although in some individuals, stress, alcohol consumption, specific foods, and oral contraceptives can trigger the cerebral vessels to constrict, causing vascular headaches.

While vitamin B_2, also known as riboflavin, isn't yet a household word in treating these painful headaches, it soon could be. In a recent study using high amounts of vitamin B_2 (400 mg per day), researchers found that the vitamin helps prevent migraines and lessens migraine symptoms in the majority of sufferers.

CONDITIONS AND DOSES

FIBROCYSTIC DISEASE

❒ **Symptoms:** Benign breast disease, chronic cystic mastitis, lumpy breasts, and mammary dysplasia are all names for fibrocystic disease, a condition characterized by one or more lumps in one or both breasts. These lumps may or may not be painful and may be accompanied by greenish or straw-colored discharge from the nipples. Unlike malignant tumors, these benign lumps are actually cysts, fluid-filled sacs that tend to get bigger toward the end of the menstrual cycle, when the body retains more fluid. Some cysts can be tiny, others can be the size of an egg. It isn't known exactly what causes fibrocystic disease, although an imbalance of ovarian hormones are believed to play a role. The disease occurs mainly in women between the ages of 25 and 50 and usually disappears with menopause.

❒ How Vitamin B_6 Can Help: **Two British studies have found vitamin B_6 helpful** in reducing fibrocystic symptoms. Vitamin B_6 is a diuretic which keeps breast tissue from retaining extra fluid. The vitamin has also been shown in animal studies to reduce the effects of excess estrogen, which has been linked to fibrocystic disease.

❏ **Dosages:** Take 25 to 50 mg of vitamin B-complex once or twice a day, plus an additional 50 to 100 mg of vitamin B_6 three times a day. Mild results can be seen after one month, with more dramatic results occurring after three months. Vitamin B_6 has been shown to be safe in amounts of 200 to 500 mg per day. However, if you experience numbness in the hands or feet, stop taking the individual vitamin B_6 supplement. Lactating women should not take more than 100 mg of vitamin B_6 a day.

HYPER NO MORE

There's lots of talk these days about attention deficit disorder (ADD) or attention deficit–hyperactivity disorder (ADHD), as it's also called. The disorder, which primarily affects children, is associated with learning difficulties and lack of social skills. It is defined as age-inappropriate impulsiveness, lack of concentration, and sometimes excessive physical activity. While the cause of the condition is unknown, theories include fetal exposure to alcohol, drugs, or cigarette smoke; preconception paternal recreational drug and/or alcohol use (which can affect sperm quality); allergies; or poor diet. The majority of sufferers outgrow the condition by their late teens.

Conventional treatment for ADD is Ritalin, an amphetamine-like drug which is a stimulant in adults but often has a calming effect in children with ADD. However, many parents are concerned about using drugs on their growing children. Fortunately, vitamin B_6 has shown promise as a treatment for ADD. In a recent study of vitamin B_6 and Ritalin, both were effective at reducing ADD symptoms. Interestingly, many children with ADD have been shown to be mildly to moderately deficient in vitamin B_6. Note: Before giving your child vitamin B_6 supplements, consult a physician. Although side effects from vitamin B_6 supplements are rare, at very high levels this vitamin can damage sensory nerves, leading to numbness in the hands and feet as well as difficulty walking.

CONDITIONS AND DOSES

CERVICAL DYSPLASIA

❒ Symptoms: Sometimes, a Pap test will show a precancerous cell. If this happens to you, the medical world will diagnose you as having cervical dysplasia. The good news is that cervical dysplasia often disappears on its own. The bad news is it can stick around and lead to cancer some years later. Cervical dysplasia is an asymptomatic condition found most often in women between the ages of 25 and 35. It has been linked to sexually transmitted diseases, such as the human papillomavirus (HPV), which causes genital warts. Infection by sexually transmitted organisms may be accompanied by oxidants, which can damage cervical cell DNA. Eventually, this cellular damage can lead to cancer.

❒ **How Vitamin B$_9$ Can Help:** Recent research, including studies published in the *Journal of the American Medical Association*, the *American Journal of Obstetrics and Gynecology*, and the *American Journal of Clinical Nutrition*, have found that vitamin B$_9$ prevents cervical cells from becoming cancerous in individuals taking oral contraceptives. Vitamin B$_9$, also known as folic acid, helps the body create healthy DNA and RNA—the genetic material that controls the growth and repair of all cells. It is in this role that the vitamin helps prevent cervical cells from growing abnormally and becoming precancerous. Interestingly, research has found that folic acid did not have the same effect in individuals who are not taking oral contraceptives. Further study is required to discover why this is.

❒ **Dosages:** Take 25 to 50 mg of vitamin B-complex once or twice a day, plus 100 to 200 mcg of folic acid three times a day.

DYSMENORRHEA

❑ **Symptoms:** Mild to moderate pain during menstruation is normal and occurs when the uterus contracts to shed its temporary lining. However, sometimes the uterus contracts more than necessary, causing extreme pain. This condition is called dysmenorrhea. It is believed to be caused by excessive levels of prostaglandins. The primary symptom is strong to severe pain in the lower abdomen during menstruation (this pain may radiate to the hips, buttocks, or thighs), nausea, vomiting, diarrhea, and general aching. Other signs may include dizziness, excessive perspiration, and fatigue.

❑ **How Vitamin B_3 Can Help:** Vitamin B_3, also called niacin, has been shown to relieve menstrual cramps when taken often and in large quantities. In a study of 40 dysmenorrhea sufferers, niacin relieved symptoms in 87.5 percent of the individuals who took doses of 200 mg a day during the menstrual cycle, and an additional 100 mg every two to three hours while experiencing menstrual cramps. Niacin improves blood circulation, and it is theorized that uterine muscles become relaxed when nourished with a strong supply of fresh blood. **Note:** Painful periods do not always indicate dysmenorrhea. In some cases they signal an underlying disease, such as endometriosis. If you suffer from painful periods, please see your physician.

❑ **Dosages:** Take 25 to 50 mg of vitamin B-complex once or twice a day, plus an additional 100 mg of niacin three to five times a day during menstruation. Note: Dosages of niacin over 50 to 100 mg can cause temporary flushing in some individuals. Taking more than 500 mg daily for several months at a time may cause liver damage. For that reason, people with hepatitis or other liver disease should consult a doctor before taking large amounts of niacin.

CONDITIONS AND DOSES

MENOPAUSE

❒ **Symptoms:** Menopause is not an illness but a natural condition that occurs when the ovaries no longer produce enough estrogen to stimulate the lining of the uterus and vagina properly. Simply put, menopause is when women no longer menstruate or get pregnant. It generally occurs somewhere between the ages of 40 and 60. One of the most famous signs of menopause is the hot flash, a sudden reddening of the face accompanied by a feeling of intense warmth. Other common symptoms include depressed mood, fluid retention, headache, insomnia, irritability, nervousness, night sweats, painful intercourse, rapid heartbeat, susceptibility to bladder problems, thinning of vaginal tissues, vaginal dryness, and weight gain. It should be noted that some women experience few symptoms, while still other encounter none at all.

❒ **How Vitamin B_6 and Vitamin B_9 Can Help:** The traditional "remedy" for menopause is hormone replacement therapy. This optional treatment uses synthetic hormones to elevate progesterone and estrogen to their premenopausal levels. The B-complex vitamins are helpful regardless of whether a woman undergoes or forgoes hormone replacement therapy. However, these vitamins don't help menopausal symptoms per se, but instead target heart disease and stroke, two illnesses that are prevalent among menopausal women. Research has shown that in menopausal women, both vitamin B_6 (pyridoxine) and vitamin B_9 (folic acid) reduce body levels of homocysteine, a naturally occurring amino acid that has been implicated in coronary artery disease and stroke.

❐ **Dosages:** Take 25 to 50 mg of vitamin B-complex once or twice a day, plus an additional 2 mg of vitamin B_6 once or twice a day, and an additional 180 mcg of vitamin B_9 once or twice a day.

PREMENSTRUAL SYNDROME

❐ **Symptoms:** Premenstrual syndrome, popularly known as PMS, is a predictable pattern of physical and emotional changes that occurs in some women just before menstruation. Symptoms range from barely noticeable to extreme and can include abdominal swelling, anxiety, bloating, breast soreness, clumsiness, depressed mood, difficulty concentrating, fatigue, fluid retention, headaches, irritability, lethargy, skin eruptions, sleep disturbances, swollen hands and feet, and weight gain. While it is not known exactly what causes the condition, theories include hormonal, nutritional, and psychological factors.

❐ **How Vitamin B_6 Can Help:** Vitamin B_6 has been shown in animal studies to reduce the effects of estrogen; excess estrogen is believed to be responsible for PMS symptoms. Human studies have shown that when taken for several months, large amounts of vitamin B_6 help relieve symptoms of PMS.

❐ **Dosages:** Take 25 to 50 mg of vitamin B-complex once or twice a day, plus an additional 50 to 100 mg of vitamin B_6 three times a day. Mild results can be seen after one month, with more dramatic results occurring after three months. Vitamin B_6 has been shown to be safe in amounts of 200 to 500 mg per day. However, if you experience numbness in the hands or feet, stop taking the individual vitamin B_6 supplement. Lactating women should not take more than 100 mg of vitamin B_6 a day.

ALTERNATIVE HEALTH STRATEGIES

Herbs, vitamins, minerals—of course these contribute to good health. But creating general well-being involves more than simply taking supplements. Good health has to do with various quality-of-life issues that can aggravate or cause stress, thus harming health. Here are some additional ways to help keep yourself well.

Improve Your Eating Habits

Here are the five main eating strategies people follow; consider finding the most healthful one that works with your lifestyle.

- **OMNIVOROUS**
- **PISCATORIAL**
- **MACROBIOTIC**
- **VEGAN**
- **VEGETARIAN**

Get More Exercise

Whether it's walking or weightlifting, exercise can help you feel better. Try any of these types:

- **STRETCHING**
- **AEROBICS**
- **STRENGTH TRAINING**

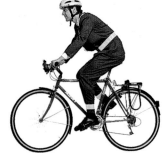

Simple Ways To Ease Stress

In addition to exercise and healthful eating, here are some more techniques—old and new—for easing stress and increasing relaxation.

- GET ENOUGH SLEEP
- MEDITATE REGULARLY
- GIVE UP JUNK FOOD
- ADOPT A PET
- SURROUND YOURSELF WITH SUPPORTIVE PEOPLE
- LIMIT YOUR EXPOSURE TO CHEMICALS
- TAKE YOUR VITAMINS
- ENJOY YOURSELF

ONE-MINUTE STRESS REDUCER

Stress is one of the top health hazards we face today. Unfortunately, it's impossible to go through life without the irritations that make us tense. Fortunately, there *is* something you can do to minimize their power to aggravate you. It's called deep breathing, and it can be done anywhere and anytime you need to calm and center yourself. Here's how to do it:

1. Inhale deeply through your nose.
2. Hold your breath for up to three seconds, then exhale through your mouth.
3. Continue as needed.

Deep breathing pulls a person's attention away from a given stressor and refocuses it on his or her breath. This type of breathing is not only comforting (thanks to its rhythmic quality), but also has been shown to lower rapid pulse and shallow respiration—two temporary symptoms of stress.

GET MOVING

Ask medical experts to name one stay-young strategy and there's a good chance "exercise" will be the answer. And with good reason. Exercise, whether a gentle walk around the block or a full-tilt weight-lifting session, strengthens the heart, lowers the body's resting heart rate, builds muscles, boosts circulation to the body and the brain, revs up the metabolism, and burns calories. All of which can keep a person looking and feeling his or her best. To be effective, exercise must be performed several times a week. Aim for at least three sessions. However, there's more than one kind of exercise. For optimum health, try a combination of aerobic exercise and strength training. And don't forget to stretch before and after each workout!

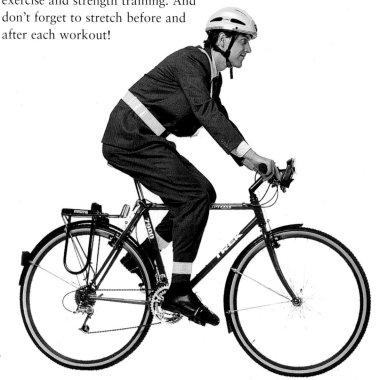

STRETCHING

❒ **What It Is:** Any movement that stretches muscles. Examples include bending at the waist and touching the toes, sitting with legs outstretched in front of you, and rolling your neck. Stretch for eight to twelve minutes before every workout and again after you exercise.

❒ **Why It's Important:** Muscles act like springs. If a muscle is short and tight, it loses the ability to absorb shock. The less shock a muscle can absorb, the more strain there is on the joints. Thus, stretching maintains flexibility, which in turn prevents injuries. Because we often lose our regular range of motion with age, stretching is especially important for older adults to prevent sprains, strains and falls.

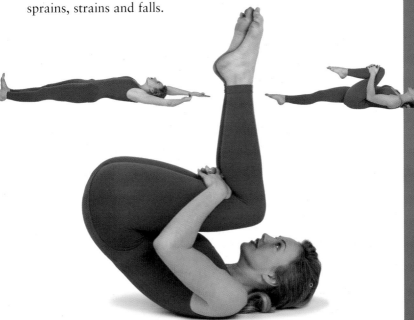

GET MOVING

AEROBICS

❒ **What It Is:** Any activity that uses large muscle groups, is maintained continuously for 15 minutes or more, and is rhythmic in nature. Examples include aerobic dance, jogging, skating, and walking. Ideally, you should aim for three to six aerobic workouts per week.

❒ **Why It's Important:** Aerobic exercise trains the heart, lungs, and cardiovascular system to process and deliver oxygen more quickly and efficiently to every part of the body. As the heart muscle becomes stronger and more efficient, a larger amount of blood can be pumped with each stroke. Fewer strokes are then required to rapidly transport oxygen to all parts of the body.

STRENGTH TRAINING

❑ **What It Is:** Any activity that improves the condition of your muscles by making repeated movements against a force. Examples include lifting large or small weights, sit-ups, stair-stepping, and isometrics.

❑ **Why It's Important:** Strength training makes it easier to move heavy loads, whether they require carrying, pushing, pulling or lifting, as well as to participate in sports that require strength. The exercises are of various kinds. Some require changing the length of the muscle while maintaining the level of tension, others involve using special equipment to vary the tension in the muscles, and some entail contracting a muscle while maintaining its length.

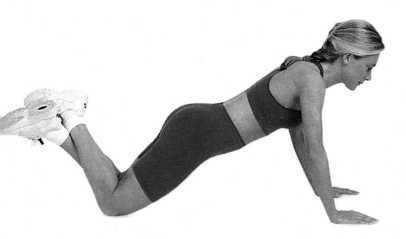

EATING SMART

A balanced diet is the foundation of good health. For proof, just read the numerous medical studies that link healthful eating with disease prevention and disease reversal. These same studies connect high fat intake, high sodium consumption, and diets with too much protein to numerous illnesses, including cancer, cardiovascular diseases, diverticular diseases, hypertension, and heart disease. But what exactly is a balanced diet? Generally speaking, it is a diet comprised of carbohydrates, dietary fiber, fat, protein, water, 13 vitamins, and 20 minerals. More specifically, it is a diet built around a wide variety of fruits, legumes, whole grains, and vegetables. Alcohol, animal protein, high-fat foods, high-sodium foods, highly-sugared foods, sodas, and processed foods are consumed sparingly, if at all.

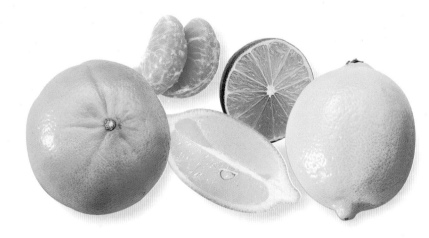

OMNIVOROUS

❑ **On the Menu:** Plant-based foods, dairy products, eggs, fish, seafood, red meats, organ meats, poultry.

❑ **Foods That Are Avoided:** None. Everything is fair game.

❑ **How Healthy Is It?** It depends. Someone who eats eggs, poultry or meat every day, chooses refined snacks over whole foods, and gets only one or two daily servings of fruits and vegetables will not be as healthy as a person who limits meat (the general dietary term for any "flesh foods," including poultry and fish) to two or three times a week, chooses water over soft drinks, and gets the recommended five or more daily servings of fruits and vegetables. Complaints about traditional omnivorous diets revolve around the diet's high level of cholesterol and saturated fat (found in animal-based foods), which increases one's risk of cancer, diabetes, heart disease, and obesity. However, an omnivorous diet can be a healthful one, provided thoughtful choices are made. To keep cholesterol and saturated fat to a minimum and nutrients to a maximum, eat five or more daily servings of fruits and vegetables, choose whole grains over refined grains, enjoy daily legume or soyfood protein sources, and limit the use of animal foods.

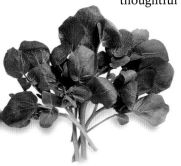

EATING SMART

MACROBIOTIC

❒ **On the Menu:** Plant-based foods, fish, very limited amounts of salt.

❒ **Foods That Are Avoided:** Dairy products, eggs, foods with artificial ingredients, hot spices, mass-produced foods, organ meats, peppers, potatoes, poultry, red meats, shellfish, warm drinks, refined foods.

❒ **How Healthy Is It?** Macrobiotics is based on a system created inn the early 1900s by Japanese philosopher George Ohsawa. The diet consists of 50 percent whole grains, 20 to 30 percent vegetables, and 5 to 10 percent beans, sea vegetables, and soy foods. The remainder of the diet is composed of white-meat fish, fruits, and nuts. The diet's low amounts of saturated fat, absence of processed foods, and emphasis on high-fiber foods, such as whole grains and vegetables, may promote cardiovascular health. Because soy and sea vegetables contain cancer-fighting compounds, macrobiotics is often recommended to help treat cancer. However, critics worry that the diet's limited variety of food can leave followers lacking in certain vitamins and important cancer-fighting phytonutrients.

50

PISCATORIAL

❑ **On the Menu:** Plant-based foods, dairy products, eggs, fish, seafood.

❑ **Foods That Are Avoided:** Red meats, organ meats, poultry.

❑ **How Healthy Is It?** Like an omnivorous diet, a piscatorial diet is as healthy as a person makes it. Individuals who eat high-fat and highly processed foods, fail to get the recommended daily number of vegetables and fruits, and eschew whole grains for processed grains will not enjoy optimum health. That said, individuals who are conscientious about eating a balanced, varied diet, and who limit fish and seafood intake to two or three times per week, can expect a lower risk of heart disease. Since many oily fish contain omega-3 fatty acids, eating oily fish in moderation has been found to help lower blood cholesterol. Be aware, however, that oily saltwater fish, such as shark, swordfish and tuna, have been found to carry mercury in their tissues; many health authorities recommend eating these varieties no more than once or twice a week. Also, due to overfishing, many fish species are now threatened, including bluefin tuna, Pacific perch, Chilean sea bass, Chinook salmon, and swordfish. For additional information on endangered fish, visit the University of Michigan's Endangered Species Update at www.umich.edu/~esuupdate, or the Fish and Wildlife Information Exchange at http://fwie.fe.vt.edu.

EATING SMART

VEGAN

❑ **On the Menu:** Plant-based foods.

❑ **Foods That Are Avoided:** Dairy, eggs, fish, seafood, red meats, organ meats, poultry. Also avoided are foods made by animals or processed with animal parts, such as gelatin, honey, marshmallows made with animal gelatin, white sugar processed with bone char.

❑ **How Healthy Is It?** A vegan (pronounced VEE-gun) diet can be extremely healthy. Like the vegetarian diet, a vegan diet has been shown by numerous studies to lower blood pressure and prevent heart disease. In addition, the high fiber intake cuts one's risk of diverticular disease and colon cancer. Yet because vegans do not eat dairy products or eggs, they must be more conscientious than vegetarians about either eating plant foods with vitamin B_{12} and vitamin D, or taking supplements of these nutrients.

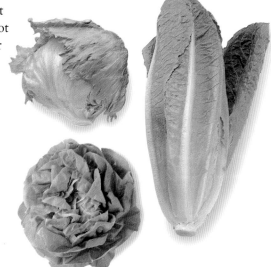

VEGETARIAN

❐ **On the Menu:** Plant-based foods, dairy, eggs.

❐ **Foods That Are Avoided:** Fish, gelatin, seafood, red meats, organ meats, poultry.

❐ **How Healthy Is It?** A vegetarian diet can be very healthy when done right. Fortunately, this isn't hard. Dietary science has debunked theories of "protein combining" popular in the 1960s and 1970s, leaving today's vegetarians to worry only about eating a wide variety of whole foods, including beans, fruits, grains, low-fat dairy products, nuts, soy foods, and vegetables. A varied daily diet insures enough protein, calcium, and other nutrients for vegetarians of all ages, including children, pregnant individuals, and the elderly. A well-chosen vegetarian eating plan has been shown by numerous studies to lower blood pressure, decrease one's risk of breast cancer, and prevent heart disease. In addition, the diet's high fiber levels cut the risk of diverticular disease and colon cancer.

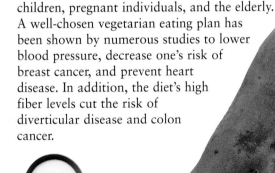

NUTRIENT KNOW-HOW

Vitamins and minerals are known collectively as nutrients. Name a body function, whether carbohydrate metabolism, nerve cell replication, or wound healing, and you'll find one or more of these nutrients at work. The best place to look for vitamins and minerals? In the food you eat every day. Indeed, if you eat a well-balanced diet there's a good chance you'll get all the nutrients your body needs. But if you are ill, pregnant, eat an inadequate diet, drink more than two alcoholic or caffeinated drinks per day,

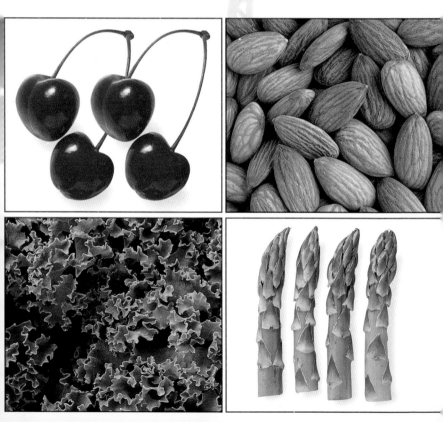

are under stress, are taking certain medications, or have difficulty absorbing certain nutrients, you may need to supplement your diet with one or more vitamins or minerals. Supplements generally come in tablet and capsule form, although some health food stores also carry liquid supplements. Whichever form you choose, doses are measured by weight in milligrams (mg); in micrograms (mcg); or in the universal standard known as international units (IU).

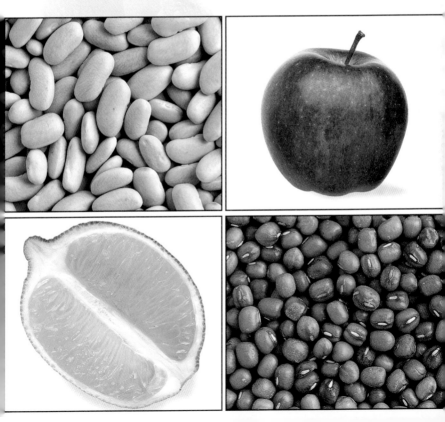

VITAMIN A

(beta carotene, retinol)

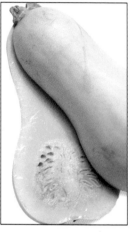

What It Does: Vitamin A is found in two forms: performed vitamin A, known as retinol, and provitamin A, called beta carotene. Retinol is found only in foods of animal origin. Beta carotene, a carotenoid, is a pigment found in plants. Beta carotene has a slight nutritional edge, boasting antioxidant properties and the ability to help lower harmful cholesterol levels. Regardless of the form, vitamin A is essential for good vision; promotes healthy skin, hair, and mucous membranes; stimulates wound healing; and is necessary for proper development of bones and teeth.

Recommended Daily Allowance: Men, 5,000 IU (or 3 mg beta carotene); women, 4,000 IU (or 2.4 mg beta carotene).

Food Sources: Orange and yellow fruits and vegetables, dark green leafy vegetables, whole milk, cream, butter, organ meats.

Toxic Dosage: When taken in excess of 10,000 IU daily, prolonged use of vitamin A supplements can cause abdominal pain, amenorrhea, dry skin, enlarged liver or spleen, hair loss, headaches, itching, joint pain, nausea, vision problems, vomiting.

Enemies: Antibiotics, cholesterol-lowering drugs, heavy laxative use.

Deficiency Symptoms: Because vitamin A is fat-soluble, it is stored in the body's fat for a long time, making deficiency uncommon. However, deficiency symptoms include dryness of the conjunctiva and cornea, frequent colds, insomnia, night blindness, reproductive difficulties, respiratory infections.

VITAMIN B_1

(thiamine)

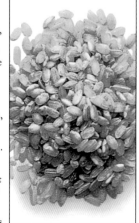

What It Does: Maintains normal nervous system functioning, helps metabolize carbohydrates, proteins, and fats; assists in blood formation and circulation; optimizes cognitive activity and brain function; regulates the body's appetite; protects the body from the degenerative effects of alcohol consumption, environmental pollution, and smoking.

Minimum Recommended Daily Allowance: Men, 1.5 mg; women, 1.1 mg.

Food Sources: Brewer's yeast, broccoli, brown rice, egg yolks, fish, legumes, peanuts, peas, pork, prunes, oatmeal, raisins, rice bran, soybeans, wheat germ, whole grains.

Toxic Dosage: There is no know toxicity level for vitamin B_1.

Enemies: Antibiotics, a diet high in simple carbohydrates, heavy physical exertion, oral contraceptives, sulfa drugs.

Deficiency Symptoms: Appetite loss, confusion, fatigue, heart arrhythmia, nausea, mood swings. Severe deficiency can lead to beriberi, a crippling disease characterized by convulsions, diarrhea, edema, gastrointestinal problems, heart failure, mental confusion, nerve damage, paralysis, severe weight loss.

VITAMIN B₂

(riboflavin, vitamin G)

What It Does: Helps metabolize carbohydrates, fats, and proteins; allows skin, nail, and hair tissues to utilize oxygen; aids in red blood cell formation and antibody production; promotes cell respiration; maintains proper nerve function, eyes, and adrenal glands.

Minimum Recommended Daily Allowance: Men, 1.7 mg; women, 1.3 mg; pregnant women, 1.6 mg.

Food Sources: Cheese, egg yolks, fish, legumes, milk, poultry, spinach, whole grains, yogurt.

Toxic Dosage: There is no known toxicity level for this vitamin, although nervousness and rapid heartbeat have been reported with daily dosages of 10 mg.

Enemies: Alcohol, oral contraceptives, strenuous exercise.

Deficiency Symptoms: Cracks at the corners of the mouth, dermatitis, dizziness, hair loss, insomnia, itchy or burning eyes, light sensitivity, mouth sores, impaired thinking, inflammation of the tongue, rashes.

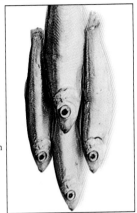

VITAMIN B₅

(pantothenic acid)

What It Does: Helps produce adrenal hormones, antibodies, and various neurotransmitters; reduces skin inflammation; speeds healing of wounds; helps convert food to energy.

Minimum Recommended Daily Allowance: 4 mg.

Food Sources: Beef, eggs, beans, brown rice, corn, lentils, mushrooms, nuts, peas, pork, saltwater fish, sweet potatoes.

Toxic Dosages: There is no known toxicity level for this vitamin; however, doses above 10 mg can cause diarrhea in some individuals.

Deficiency Symptoms: Vitamin B₅ deficiency is extremely rare and is likely to occur only with starvation.

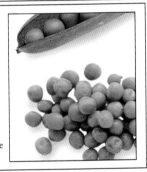

VITAMIN B₆

(pyridoxine)

What It Does: Involved in more bodily functions than nearly any other nutrient. It helps the body metabolize carbohydrates, fats and proteins; supports immune function; helps build red blood cells; assists in transmission of nerve impulses; maintains the body's sodium and potassium balance; helps synthesize RNA and DNA.

Minimum Recommended Daily Allowance: Men, 2 mg; women, 1.6 mg; pregnant women, 2.2 mg.

Food Sources: Avocados, bananas, beans, blackstrap molasses, brown rice, carrots, corn, fish, nuts, sunflower seeds.

Toxic Dosage: Levels of 2,000 to 5,000 mg can cause numbness in the hands and feet, and insomnia.

Deficiency Symptoms: Vitamin B₆ deficiency is rare. Symptoms include depression, fatigue, flaky skin, headaches, insomnia, irritability, muscle weakness, nausea.

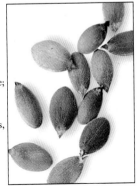

VITAMIN B₁₂

(cobalamin)

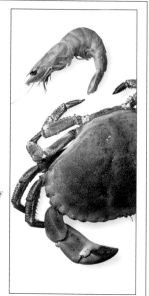

What It Does: Regulates formation of red blood cells, helps the body utilize iron; converts carbohydrates, fats, and proteins into energy; aids in cellular formation and cellular longevity; prevents nerve damage; maintains fertility; promotes normal growth.

Minimum Recommended Daily Allowance: Adults, 2 mg; pregnant women, 2.2 mg.

Food Sources: Brewer's yeast, dairy products, eggs, organ meats, seafood, sea vegetables, tempeh.

Toxic Dosage: There is no known toxicity level for vitamin B₁₂.

Enemies: Anticoagulant drugs, anti gout medication, potassium supplements.

Deficiency Symptoms: While deficiency is rare, individuals who do not eat animal products are at risk unless they fortify their diets with plant-sources such as brewer's yeast and sea vegetables. Symptoms include back pain, body odor, constipation, dizziness, fatigue, moodiness, numbness and tingling in the arms and legs, ringing in the ears, muscle weakness, tongue inflammation, weight loss. Severe deficiency can lead to pernicious anemia, characterized by abdominal pain, stiffness in the arms and legs, a tendency to bleed, yellowish cast to the skin, permanent nerve damage, death.

VITAMIN C

(ascorbic acid)

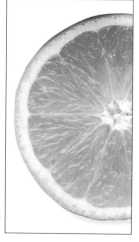

What It Does: Protects against pollution and infection, enhances immunity; aids in growth and repair of both bone and tissue by helping the body produce collagen; maintains adrenal gland function; helps the body absorb iron; aids in production of antistress hormones; reduces cholesterol levels; lowers high blood pressure; prevents artherosclerosis.

Minimum Recommended Daily Allowance: Adults, 60 mg; pregnant women, 70 mg.

Food Sources: Berries, cantaloupe, citrus fruits, broccoli, leafy greens, mangoes, papayas, peppers, persimmons, pineapple, tomatoes.

Toxic Dosage: Doses larger than 10,000 mg can cause diarrhea, stomach irritation, or increased kidney stone formation. **Enemies:** Alcohol, analgesics, antidepressants, anticoagulants, oral contraceptives, smoking, steroids.

Deficiency Symptoms: Bleeding gums, easy bruising, fatigue, reduced resistance to colds and other infections, slow healing of wounds, weight loss. Severe deficiency can lead to scurvy, a sometimes-fatal disease characterized by aching bones, muscle weakness, and swollen and bleeding gums.

VITAMIN D

(calciferol, ergosterol)

What It Does: Helps the body utilize calcium and phosphorus; promotes normal development of bones and teeth; assists in thyroid function; maintains normal blood clotting; helps regulate heartbeat, nerve function, and muscle contraction.

Minimum Recommended Daily Allowance: Adults, 200 IU (5 mcg); pregnant women, 400 IU (10 mcg).

Food Sources: Dandelion greens, dairy products, eggs, fatty saltwater fish, parsley, sweet potatoes, vegetable oils.

Toxic Dosage: Daily doses higher than 400 IU can lead to raised blood calcium levels and calcium deposits of the heart, liver, and kidney.

Enemies: Antacids, cholesterol-lowering drugs, cortisone drugs.

Deficiency Symptoms: The body naturally manufactures about 200 IU of vitamin D when exposed to ten minutes of ultraviolet light, making deficiency rare. Symptoms include bone weakening, diarrhea, insomnia, muscle twitches, vision disturbances. Severe deficiency can lead to rickets, a disease that results in bone defects such as bowlegs and knock-knees.

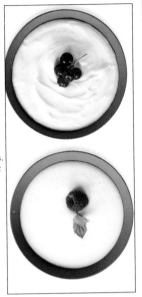

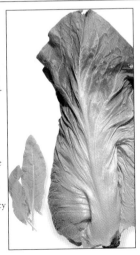

VITAMIN E

(tocopherol)

What It Does: Prevents unstable molecules known as free radicals from damaging cells and tissue; accelerates wound healing; protects lung tissue from inhaled pollutants; aids in functioning of the immune system; endocrine system, and sex glands; improves circulation; promotes normal blood clotting.

Minimum Recommended Daily Allowance: Men, 15 IU (10 mg); women, 12 IU (8 mg); pregnant women, 15 IU (10 mg).

Food Sources: Avocados, dark green leafy vegetables, eggs, legumes, nuts, organ meats, seafood, seeds, soybeans.

Toxic Dosage: Although there is no established toxicity level of vitamin E, the vitamin has blood-thinning properties; individuals who are taking anticoagulant medications or have clotting deficiencies should avoid vitamin E.

Enemies: High temperatures and overcooking reduce vitamin E levels in food.

Deficiency Symptoms: Vitamin E deficiency is rare. Deficiency symptoms include fluid retention, infertility, miscarriage, muscle degeneration.

CALCIUM

What It Does: Necessary for the growth and maintenance of bones, teeth, and healthy gums; maintains normal blood pressure normal; may reduce risk of heart disease; enables muscles, including the heart, to contract; is essential for normal blood clotting; needed for proper nerve impulse transmission; maintains connective tissue; helps prevent rickets and osteoporosis.

Minimum Recommended Daily Allowance: Adults, 800 mg; pregnant women, 1,200 mg.

Food Sources: Asparagus, cruciferous vegetables, dairy products, dark leafy vegetables, figs, legumes, nuts, oats, prunes, salmon with bones, sardines with bones, seeds, soybeans, tempeh, tofu.

Toxic Dosage: Daily intake of 2,000 mg or more can lead to constipation, calcium deposits in the soft tissue, urinary tract infections, and possible interference with the body's absorption of zinc.

Enemies: Alcohol, caffeine, excessive sugar intake, high-protein diet, high sodium intake, inadequate levels of vitamin D, soft drinks containing phosphorous.

Deficiency Symptoms: Aching joints, brittle nails, eczema, elevated blood cholesterol. heart palpitations, hypertension, insomnia, muscle cramps, nervousness, pallor, tooth decay.

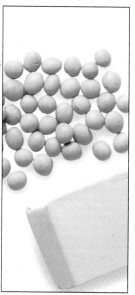

IRON

What It Does: Aids in the production of hemoglobin (the protein in red blood cells that transports oxygen from the lungs to the body's tissue) and myoglobin (a protein that provides extra fuel to muscles during exertion); helps maintain healthy immune system; is important for growth.

Minimum Recommended Daily Allowance: Men, 10 mg; women, 15 mg; pregnant women, 30 mg.

Food Sources: Beef, blackstrap molasses, brewer's yeast, dark green vegetables, dried fruit, legumes, nuts, organ meats, sea vegetables, seeds, soybeans, tempeh, whole grains.

Toxic Dosage: Iron should not be taken in excess of 35 mg daily without a doctor's recommendation. In high doses, iron cam cause diarrhea, dizziness, fatigue, headaches, stomach-aches, weakened pulse. Excess iron inhibits the absorption of phosphorus and vitamin E, interferes with immune function, and has been associated with cancer, cirrhosis, heart disease.

Enemies: Antacids, caffeine, tetracycline, iron absorption, excessive menstrual bleeding, long-term illness, an ulcer.

Deficiency Symptoms: Anemia, brittle hair, difficulty swallowing, dizziness, fatigue, hair loss, irritability, nervousness, pallor, ridges on the nails, sensitivity to cold, slowed mental reactions.

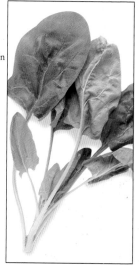

MAGNESIUM

What It Does: Plays a role in formation of bone; protects arterial linings from stress caused by sudden blood pressure; helps body metabolize carbohydrates and minerals; assists in building proteins; helps maintain healthy bones and teeth; reduces one's risk of developing osteoporosis.

Minimum Recommended Daily Allowance: Men, 350 mg; women, 280 mg; pregnant women, 320 mg.

Food Sources: Apples, apricots, avocados, bananas, blackstrap molasses, brewer's yeast. brown rice, cantaloupe, dairy products, figs, garlic, green leafy vegetables, legumes, nuts.

Toxic Dosage: Daily doses over 3,000 mg can lead to diarrhea, fatigue, muscle weakness, and in extreme cases, severely depressed heart rate and blood pressure, shallow breathing, loss of reflexes and coma.

Enemies: Alcohol, diuretics, high-fat intake, high-protein diet.

Deficiency Symptoms: Though deficiency is rare, symptoms include disorientation, heart palpitations, listlessness, muscle weakness.

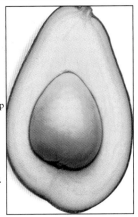

POTASSIUM

What It Does: Maintains a healthy nervous system and regular heart rhythm; helps prevent stroke; aids in proper muscle contractions; controls the body's water balance; assists chemical reactions within cells; aids in the transmission of electrochemical impulses; maintains stable blood pressure; required for protein synthesis, carbohydrate metabolism, and insulin secretion by the pancreas.

Minimum Recommended Daily Allowance: Adults, 2,000 mg.

Food Sources: Apricots, avocados, bananas, blackstrap molasses, brewer's yeast, brown rice, citrus fruits, dairy.

Toxic Dosage: Should not be taken in excess of 18 grams.

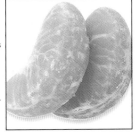

Enemies: Diarrhea, diuretics, caffeine use, heavy perspiration, kidney disorders, tobacco use.

Deficiency Symptoms: Chills, dry skin, constipation, depression, diminished reflexes, edema, headaches, insatiable thirst, fluctuations in heartbeat, nervousness, respiratory distress.

ZINC

What It Does: Contributes to a wide range of bodily processes. Aids in cell respiration; assists in bone development; helps energy metabolism, promotes wound healing; regulates heart rate and blood pressure; helps liver remove toxic substances, such as alcohol, from the body.

Minimum Recommended Daily Allowance: Adults, 15 mg; pregnant women, 30 mg.

Food Sources: Brewer's yeast, cheese, egg yolks, lamb, legumes, mushrooms, nuts, organ meats, sea food, sea vegetables, seeds.

Toxic Dosage: Do not take more than 100. mg of zinc daily. In doses this high, zinc can depress the immune system.

Deficiency Symptoms: Appetite loss, dermatitis, fatigue, impaired wound healing, loss of taste, white streaks on the nails.

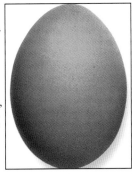

INDEX

ABOUT THE AUTHOR

Stephanie Pedersen is a writer and editor who specializes in the area of health. Her articles have appeared in numerous publications, including *American Woman, Sassy, Teen, Weight Watchers* and *Woman's World*. She has also co-written *What Your Cat is Trying to Tell You: A Head-to-Tail Guide to Your Cat's Symptoms and Their Solutions* and *What Your Dog is Trying to Tell You: A Head-to-Tail Guide to Your Dog's Symptoms and Their Solutions,* both published by St. Martin's Press. She currently resides in New York City.

Picture Credits: Steve Gorton, David Murray, Dave King, Martin Norris, Philip Gatward, Andy Crawford, Philip Dowell, Clive Streeter, Peter Chadwick, Tim Ridley, Andrew Whittack, Martin Cameron

DORLING KINDERSLEY PUBLISHING, INC.
www.dk.com

Published in the United States by
Dorling Kindersley Publishing, Inc.
95 Madison Avenue • New York, New York 10016

Editorial Director: LaVonne Carlson
Editors: Nancy Burke, Barbara Minton, Connie Robinson
Designer: Carol Wells
Cover Designer: Gus Yoo

Library of Congress Cataloging-in-Publication Data is available upon request.
ISBN: 0-7894-5195-6